THIS BOOK BELONGS TO

_____

A GIFT FROM

_____

_____DATE_____

Comments:_____
_____
_____
_____
_____

TOWARD BETTER DAYS

Author

Martha I. Clyburn
DBA: Expressions From Heart and Hills
Marthaclyburn.com
Marthaclyburn1@gmail.com

1st printing 2010   2nd printing 2019

Introduction

Former First Lady Rosalynn Carter said, "There are only four kinds of people in the world; those who have been caregivers, those who currently are caregivers, those who will be caregivers, those who will need caregivers."

It is a life changing occurrence for everyone when someone close to you becomes ill or incapacitated. 80% of the care needed by older adults is provided by a family member or friend; 80% of caregivers provide care seven days a week for an average of four hours a day; 64% of caregivers are employed; the average age of caregivers is 46; one-third of caregivers are the sole caregiver for their loved one; caregivers experiencing stress and strain have a 63% higher risk of death. *Being a caregiver has an tremendous impact on all phases of your life and those close to you.*

I have been through this maze of life changing emotions and experiences five times as a caregiver to loved ones. During the times when I was a caregiver I came to realize the need for and the benefit of a central place to keep medical and other important information. Thus, I created this user friendly informational workbook, "Toward Better Days"

I designed and used forms similar to those in this book to help me track concerns, progress, visitors, family information and other details. <u>Some of these forms you will want to adapt to your own needs and/or make multiple copies of mine.</u> The ones in this book will provide basic information and suggestions and can be a reminder of what you may need to do.

This information proved helpful for family and friends who wanted to review the patient's condition and treatments, as well as for medical personnel who needed to know any changes in condition, comments from the caregiver, medications/dosages, etc. EMT's always need information readily available in order to make critical decisions on treatments.

The forms can be an asset in tracking schedules for medications, and keeping a record of important contacts, phone numbers, personal information, and health history as well as reminders for daily activities and appointments. *Being able to locate information quickly is an invaluable aid.*

When someone is ill there are many needs which unexpectedly arise. Most people are not aware of the vast number of resources for information and assistance. Some of these resources are included for your guidance.

The practical information in this book is presented surrounded by photos, poems, and whimsy in the hopes of bringing smiles, happy memories, comforting thoughts, or a moment of escape to those in need, as well as being a useable resource.
2Included also is a guest registry with a place for comments from visitors and a record of gifts; this is a great reminder for thank you notes and follow up.

I hope this book will be a blessing to patients and caregivers and will serve as a reminder of some information that everyone should have readily available.

(Though this book was written with the incapacitated and the caregiver in mind it is an excellent resource and reference for having one central place to keep important information. Everyone will have a time in their life when personal and family health history and other personal information is needed by them or by persons who need to take care of them. Having information readily available can save many hours of frustration in a crisis.)

Remember to always keep looking "Toward Better Days".

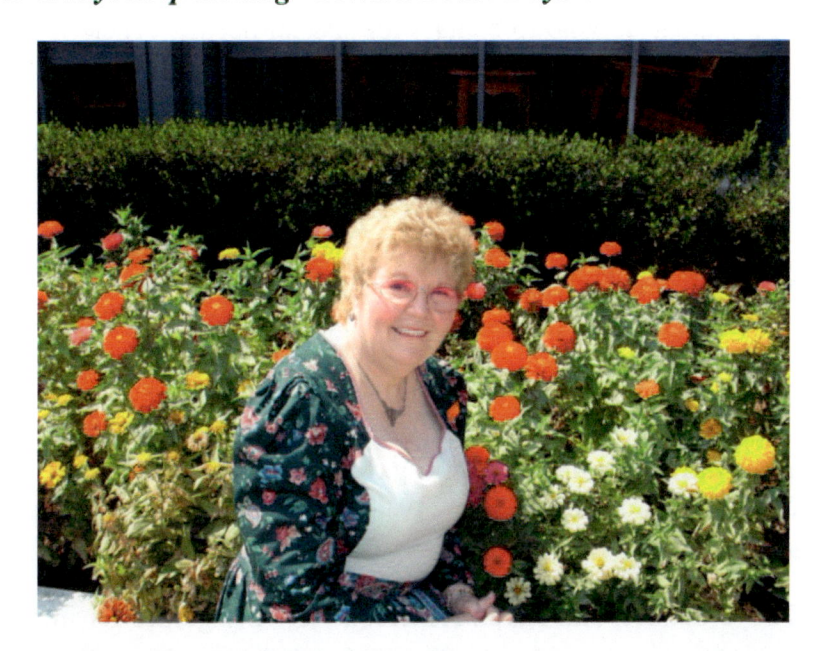

{The author, Martha I. Clyburn worked as a social worker and counselor for many years; this gave her the opportunity to work with people of all ages and conditions encompassing numerous problems. In these positions she learned about the many community services and resources which were available. She researched and designed a Community Services Directory for a county in metropolitan Atlanta, Georgia.

As a writer, photographer, and poet she has published four books, one on the crafts of the Blue Ridge Mountains for use in Adult Education classes, and one on the history of Helen, Georgia's Alpine Village, and a memoir "Why Be Normal?"
She has also written numerous articles for various publications. She is a member of the Writers' Workshop and the International Women's Writing Guild.

This book is the result of a natural progression from her social services background, her writing experiences, and her personal experiences as a caregiver.

The photos and poems included reflect her love of nature, the mountain areas of northern Georgia and North Carolina where she has lived, and other places and events which have special meaning for her.

All photos and writings are those of the author except as otherwise noted I could not have written this book without the input from so many people, most of whom remain nameless to me---doctors, nurses, hospice staff, hospital staff, social workers, chaplains, and volunteers. As a caregiver when I worked with them and talked with them I learned so much about everything from bathing a patient, to who to contact for special needs. There is much I still do not know, but I did gain a good overview of what to expect and how to deal with most needs of an incapacitated person. All of these people were dedicated and devoted to the needs of the patient and me; I could not have made it through the complications and extreme emotional stress of being a caregiver without their help and input.

A special thank you goes to the staff of Four Seasons Hospice in Hendersonville, N.C. They were a blessing to me, my loved ones and my family during the illness of two of my loved ones. To Pat, Jane, Rausey, the staff at Elizabeth House, and all the other staff of Four Seasons Hospice that crossed my path I am forever indebted.

Thanks to Ruth Price, Holley Hovermale, Millie Clements, Gretchen Hall and Toni C. Barksdale, friends and family involved in the healthcare industry, who gave me input from their perspective on important points to remember. Their information was invaluable reminding me of details that needed to be included.

Friends Elizabeth Wallrich, Tonya Staufer, and Karen Ackerson were my guides for improving this book. They have reviewed, edited, proofed, and reviewed again my many drafts. Their input was priceless.

My deep appreciation to life-long friend and award winning author Bill Abbott who encouraged me to keep going and offered information on the ins and outs of producing this book

Finally, this book would not have been written if not for Bill Rector, my significant other for 16 years. For ten years he gave me constant support and encouragement to publish this book. After his death I felt his presence urging me to complete this project and to make it available to others who could benefit from my knowledge.

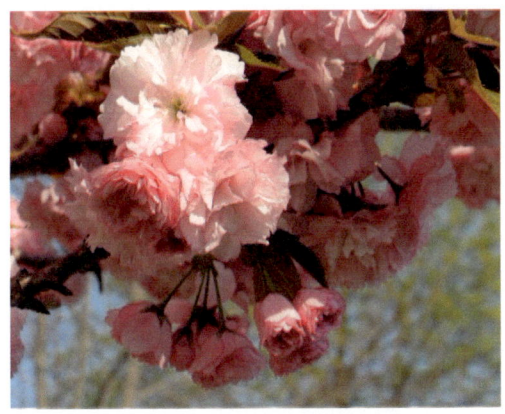

Testimonials

"I wish I had had this book when my mother was ill. I had no idea of what to expect or what I needed to do---I needed guidance. I especially wish I had had the visitor/gift register and the daily diary so I could read them now and remember."   Faye Chambers, Lawrenceville, Georgia

"As a physical therapist I can see the value of this book across various patient populations from geriatrics to pediatrics. This book gives caregivers a sense of security and control by having information documented and readily accessible when faced with decisions. What an excellent resource for families and attending medical professionals to draw from!" Dr Holley Hovermale, DPT. Rocky Ridge, Maryland

"--- anyone who has not been in this situation --- has no idea what is in store for them. --- things really came as a surprise for us. I think you are giving advice that will be helpful to many people. "   Jack Holley. Chamblee, Georgia

"Many families just have no idea where to turn when it becomes time to "care " for parents who have always made their own decisions and 'called the shots'. It is my opinion that to take charge, be preventive, is more loving than to wait for the crisis that requires changes. This guidebook can assist with such decisions."   Millie Clements, Access Millie, Inc. Home Health Care Agency. Hall County, Ga.

"I find Martha's book concise and informative and offering a one place source for any and all necessary information for caregivers. The resources and reminders are gentle and thoughtful. They offer a sense of calm and assurance for those who serve others and remind them that they matter too."   Pastor Michael S. Byrum. Hendersonville, NC.

"Family members and friends often want to know about the patient. If information is kept in this book they can easily review progress, medications, medical information and reports. This is especially important for family and friends who are relieving the primary caregiver for a time and need to be aware of circumstances, administering medications, emergency contacts, and other details of care." Jean Key, Caregiver and sitter for 35 years.

"The best time for caregivers to read this book is early in the process; this author has succeeded in her intent to provide some tools to lessen the stress and exhaustion inevitably experienced by every caregiver."   Gretchen Hall, RN, MSN, FNP, former hospice nurse and 13 year primary caregiver for husband who struggled with Alzheimer's disease.

"What a delight to see how you have turned your own experiences into a book that can benefit other caregivers: I really like the idea of the forms for sharing and compiling information. Also, since you have been a caregiver, the book has an authentic voice which I believe people will trust."   Ruth Price, Coordinator,   Park Ridge Hospital's HOPE Behavioral Health Caregiver Wellness Program. Henderson County, N. C.

The Butterfly

A man found a cocoon of a butterfly. One day a small opening appeared. He sat and watched the butterfly for several hours as it struggled to force its body through that little hole. Then it seemed to stop making any progress. It appeared as if it had gotten as far as it could and it could go no further. So the man decided to help the butterfly. He took a pair of scissors and snipped off the remaining bit of the cocoon. The butterfly then emerged easily. But it had a swollen body and small shriveled wings. The man continued to watch the butterfly because he expected that at any moment, the wings would enlarge and expand to be able to support the body. Neither happened. In fact, the butterfly spent the rest of its life crawling around with a swollen body and shriveled wings. It never was able to fly. What the man did not understand was that the restricting cocoon and the struggle required for the butterfly to get through the tiny opening were God's way of forcing fluid from the body of the butterfly into its wings so that it would be ready for flight once it achieved its freedom from the cocoon.

Sometimes struggles are exactly what we need in our lives. If God allowed us to go through our lives without any obstacles, it would cripple us. We would not be as strong as what we could have been. *We could never fly!*

Anonymous

This book is dedicated in loving memory of:

Carol Clyburn Kinsman, my sister

Martha Launius Clyburn, my mother

Bill (Pine Knot) Rector, my significant other

Lois Tomlin Rector and Ruby Cleo Stepp, my dear friends

Thankfully I was able to take care of these loved ones during their dark days of illness. This book grew out of knowledge I gained from them, the professionals who took care of them and my personal experiences during these times.
–*Martha I. Clyburn*

The Scent of the Roses
Let fate do her worst; there are relics of joy,
Bright Dreams of the past, which she cannot destroy,
Which come in the night-time of sorrow and care,
And bring back the features that joy used to wear.
Long, long be my heart with such memories filled
Like the vase in which roses have once been distilled---
You may break, you may shatter the vase if you will
But the scent of the roses will hang round it still.
Thomas Moore

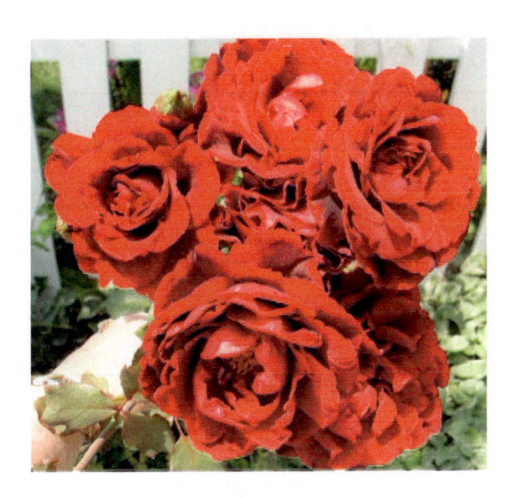

Day/Date **Visitors/Flowers/Gifts**
Messages and Get Well Wishes

Day/Date   **_Visitors/Flowers/Gifts_**
                Messages and Get Well Wishes

Day/Date   *Visitors/Flowers/Gifts*
                 Messages and Get Well Wishes

FOR THE CAREGIVER

This is probably the most challenging time of your life; there are many demands on you and many varying emotions. Situations from the past and the present collide and worrying and planning for the future (even the next day) can be an overwhelming and sometimes impossible task. Try to take each day and each crisis as it comes. You can not plan the next few minutes, hours or days.

There will probably be financial strain for you and/or your loved one. If there is a long-term health care insurance policy contact the insurance company at diagnosis; some pay for in home care. Most policies require that the family caregiver take a short course and become certified before they can be paid for care. However, some do have options for cash or for caregiver payment. Take advantage of all income benefits.

In your day to day care, try to be objective about the patient. Sometimes this means being firm, but always be firm in a loving and caring manner. If they refuse to do something which is important, walk away and try to get them to do it at a later time. However, always let the patient know they are cared about; touch them, hug them---let them feel the love.

You may want to share some of the photos, poems, or whimsy from this book with your loved one; this may encourage the incapacitated person to discuss feelings or memories or to remind them of a favorite joke or story. Do anything you can to stimulate the patient and their mind and to brighten their day.

Do not ask patients to do things which they need to do, gently **tell them what they need to do or are going to do**. (i.e. the answer will almost always be NO to any questions. Say you need to eat this, or it is time to eat, or it is time to go to the toilet, let's go to the toilet, etc. Do not ask do you want to eat or do you want to go to the toilet.) You need to decide (with professionals' help) whether you are encouraging and pushing in a positive way, or are you nagging, i.e. forcing the patient to eat more than they truly want or need, etc.

Patients, especially elderly patients, tend to be angry --- they are angry about their condition, their circumstances, their regrets of the past, their loss of hope for the future. Understand this is often a large part of the situation you will find yourself in. You must remain positive. Do not argue with them. Often they strike out at the people who care about them the most, especially the caregiver. They have no one else they can vent their anger on. Try to find out if there is a real issue making them upset. There are times when you will be very angry and/or hurt because of things that are said, but you are the one who must remain positive around the patient. If you need to cry or be angry, go outside, or go talk with a friend and vent.

Friends are a blessing for caregivers; they are invaluable at this time---just lending their ear can help you focus and gain perspective. **Caregivers can not do everything by themselves**; even mundane everyday tasks become overwhelming when you have this responsibility. ***If friends*** *offer to help, let them*. *I can not emphasize this enough*. Tell them what you need. It may be as simple as vacuuming, fixing a meal, buying groceries, picking up a prescription, or sitting with the patient so you can get out for a while and regroup your own energies and emotions or take a nap. No task is too small to help you get through the day. Friends offer because they care and they genuinely want to do something to help

If there are caregiver support groups in the area, get involved. You would be amazed what information can be gleaned from someone in a similar situation.

Talk openly with the doctors and nurses handling the care of the patient. *Ask any and all questions.* **YOU MUST BE THE ADVOCATE FOR THE PATIENT.** Patients usually do not fully comprehend information about their condition, medications, or treatments. YOU are the person who really sees what is happening. Be aware of all treatments, medicines, etc. Make notes of dates and information---a change in medication, treatments, vital signs, etc. (I was once told by a doctor in the hospital I kept better and more detailed records than the nurses and he was better able to know what was actually happening.) *Write down and date all pertinent information*.

Keep all pertinent information about the patient handy and visible. In case of emergency, medical personnel will need details on medications and dosages being given, as well as the patient's doctor and phone number. In a crisis you will need to know whether there is a DNR (Do Not Resuscitate) order or Living Will (Advanced Directive), who the emergency contacts are, if there is an Attorney in Fact for medical and/or financial purposes and who these people are and their contact numbers.

Finally, and most importantly, *take care of yourself both physically and mentally*. It is too easy and common for caregivers to not eat properly and/or not get enough rest creating health problems for them; remember, **caregivers under stress and strain have a 63% higher risk of mortality.** You can't help someone else if you are not the best you can be. Don't be ashamed to ask someone to help and let you take a nap or fix a meal for you. Try to keep some schedule for yourself---as much as the situation allows. Do something occasionally that makes you happy---find a quiet place and read, take a short trip, go shopping, take a walk in the woods, etc. **You must keep in touch with the reality of your life.**

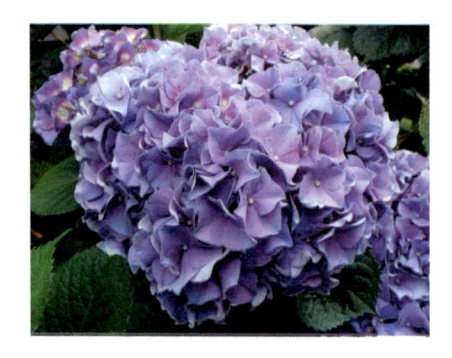

****

There may be times when you can no longer handle the situation; you may need to place your loved one in an assisted living facility or nursing home. Be careful about selecting one. Many facilities today are beautiful, but beautiful does not mean they can properly care for your loved one. Check out the facility; go often and check each shift. If you are told you need to make an appointment, skip this facility. Ask questions. If your loved one has Dementia are they protected against wandering? What quality is the food? What is the staff/patient ratio? What are the bath facilities? What are the recreation and therapy facilities? Talk to residents, you can learn a lot from them. There are many factors to consider when choosing a facility; some specialize in specific needs, be sure the facility you choose is the right one for your loved one. Start looking early so that you can make the right decision the first time; it is hard to relocate someone who is already settled.

If your loved one is in an assisted living facility or a nursing home the care giver still has responsibilities. Since you can't be there all the time you need to be aware of a number of tasks or needs:

1 Always talk with the nurse or doctor when visiting and get all updated information. Be sure to write this information down and leave it in the room for other visitors or family members that come by, and for an on-going reference of medications and the patient's improving/deteriorating condition

2 Put the patient's name on all clothes and personal items.

3 Do not leave any jewelry or large amounts of money with the patient.

4 Take photographs of the room and personal items that are there.

5 Keep a basket of "goodies" near the door for the staff. They will come by to get some and will be looking in on the patient.

6 Double check medications, reactions, timely administration of drugs.

7 Check the bed for cleanliness.

8 Be sure the call button and TV remote is where the patient can reach it.

9 Check for red spots---indications of possible bed sores or lack of cleanliness.

10 Be sure the facility has all the necessary paper work in case of an emergency (living will, DNR order, organ donation information emergency numbers of caregiver/family members, etc)

11 If the patient can not eat or drink by themselves be sure that someone

is available to help them. (I have seen staff put the tray in the room and come back later and pick it up; no one tried to feed the patient)

Remember, finances can be a big problem. File for long-term health care insurance immediately.

KEEP ALL RECEIPTS and submit them to the insurance/Medicare/Medicaid offices as soon as practical. ***KEEP COPIES OF ALL FORMS AND RECEIPTS AND LETTERS SENT TO YOUR INSURANCE COMPANIES OR MEDICARE/MEDICAID.***

Set up files for each company or organization to whom items are submitted---this is the only way to be sure items are paid, and/or you are reimbursed. Often you have to wait for one organization to pay, then submit to others (as with supplemental insurance or if two insurance policies are in force.) Don't neglect turning in insurance claims---premiums have been paid, get what money is due.

****

If your loved one is nearing death, be prepared. Go to the funeral home and make arrangements ahead of time. (In the emotional throws of a death, bad decisions can be made, funeral costs inflated or important details overlooked.). Have the burial clothes ready and take them to the funeral home.

Find out about financial arrangements and insurance.

Keep a copy of important contacts handy so calls to family, friends, and others can be made in a timely manner.

I can not say strongly enough **DO NOT WAIT UNTIL SOMEONE HAS PASSED TO START PLANNING A FUNERAL**. You as a caregiver will already be stressed and exhausted. Grief will add to your frustration and will often leave you confused and not thinking clearly. Plan ahead!!!

One of the most difficult parts of being a caregiver is when the crisis is over, by recovery or death. Don't beat up on yourself by saying maybe I didn't do enough, maybe I could have done something different, etc, etc.

Do the best you can at the time, make the best decisions you can given all the facts you know at any given time, and know in your heart and mind that is all you can do. The rest is in God's hands.

RESOURCES

There are many resources to help with problems of the incapacitated and the caregiver; this is a partial list of places to seek help. DO NOT BE AFRAID OR ASHAMED TO ASK FOR HELP. There is assistance for most any situation.
>>

A **hospital Social Worker** can be a great help. Not only can they guide you through the hospital regimen, but can offer special assistance:
1. Most hospitals have *rooms available* for the caregiver to use for sleeping or can make sleeping arrangements in the room with the ill person. Some hospitals have or can give referrals to local facilities available for caregivers or out patients at little or no cost (i.e. Ronald McDonald House.).
2. Hospitals have *chaplains* of various faiths. The Social Worker can be sure that you see the person of your choice.
3. *Legal documents* such as Living Wills, Organ Donor forms, Wills, etc. can be drawn up by the Social Worker or they will know who you should contact.
4. *Monies and special items* are sometimes available in an emergency situation.
5. Assistance with *transportation* can often be arranged. Some airlines offer special rates for persons getting medical treatment. There is an Angel Flight program. Special travel arrangements for bed bound persons or those traveling with equipment can be made. There are local ambulance services and some church groups which furnish transportation for non-emergency treatment.
6. *Child care* may be available through the hospital or community groups.

Other places to contact for information or assistance are:
- **Local Health Department**
- **State Health Department**
- **Veterans Administration**
- **Visiting Nurses Association**
- **Area Agency on Aging or Local/County Council on Aging**
- **Local Home Healthcare Agencies**
- **Local Welfare or Family and Children's Services Office**
- **Hospice**
- **Meals on Wheels**
- **Sitter Services**
- **Churches**
- **Local Respite Groups**
- **Caregiver Groups**
- **Support Groups**
- **Medical Equipment Supply Businesses**
- **Attorneys/local Bar Association**
- **Funeral Homes**

Special Organizations or support groups (local or on-line) i.e.:
American Cancer Society, Alzheimer's Association, Brain Tumor Foundation, Easter Seal Society, American Red Cross, etc. (If you don't know who to contact ask you doctor, your hospital social worker, or go on line and search for information on the particular disease or problem. Most diseases and health problems have research and/or support organizations)

The **internet** is a good source for information. You can search for information on medications, support groups, societies or organizations that focus on specific problems, treatments available, research groups and organizations, experimental treatments, hospitals that specialize in specific problems, and much more. Go to the web and search for the specific disease or problem, or go to sites such as WebMD.com, Medem.com, Dr.Koop.com, ama-assn.org/, Mayo Clinic.com, etc
Other sites which may give you information and guidance are: Family Caregiver Alliance---www.caregiver.com; The Rosalynn Carter Institute for Caregiving---www.rosalynncarter.org; Full Circle of Care---www.fullcirclecare.org; The National Council on the Aging---www.benefitscheckup.com; Friends of Residents in Long Term Care---www.forltc.org; Children of Aging Parents (CAPS)---www.caps4caregivers.org; National Mental Health Association---www.nmha.org; National Academy of Elder Law Attorneys, Inc.---www.naela.org; National Family Caregiver Support Program---www.aoa.gov/prof/aoaprog/caregiver/caregiver.asp; AARP-- www.aarp.org.

There are a number of medical sites on line. Always check several sources for information and evaluate it carefully. Discuss information with your doctor. *NEVER* change medications or treatments without discussing it with your doctor. (As few as three (3) medications cause drug interactions---some interactions may be bad, others deadly.) There are alternative treatments available for many problems, but be sure you know all the details.

If you need help yourself, or need help caring for an incapacitated person, ask your friends, relatives, church, home healthcare agencies, hospice or others. There are numerous individuals and organizations that will help clean, cook, sit, offer respite services, shop or whatever is needed. Often church groups or individuals (possibly your Habitat for Humanity) will help make the home handicap accessible.

Many items such as hospital beds, bed-side toilets, walkers, tub stools, bed wedges, wheelchairs, and many other items or equipment may be available through your insurance, Medicare, or Medicaid. Some items are approved for rental, some for purchase. Often a Certificate of Medical Necessity is required from the doctor. Some of these items need a prescription from a doctor for them to be covered. These make the patient more comfortable and help the caregiver, but **do NOT just go out and buy items**. Check with your insurance companies, your local medical equipment supplier, pharmacy or Medicare and Medicaid offices to see what is covered. There is a booklet available on Medicare services. Medicare has rules about handicap equipment: i.e. if someone is approved for a power wheel chair, they can not go back and get a regular wheel chair even though their condition may have improved. Your medical supplier should be able to help you with Medicare and Medicaid guidelines. ALWAYS ask if your supplier is an active Medicare/Medicaid supplier.

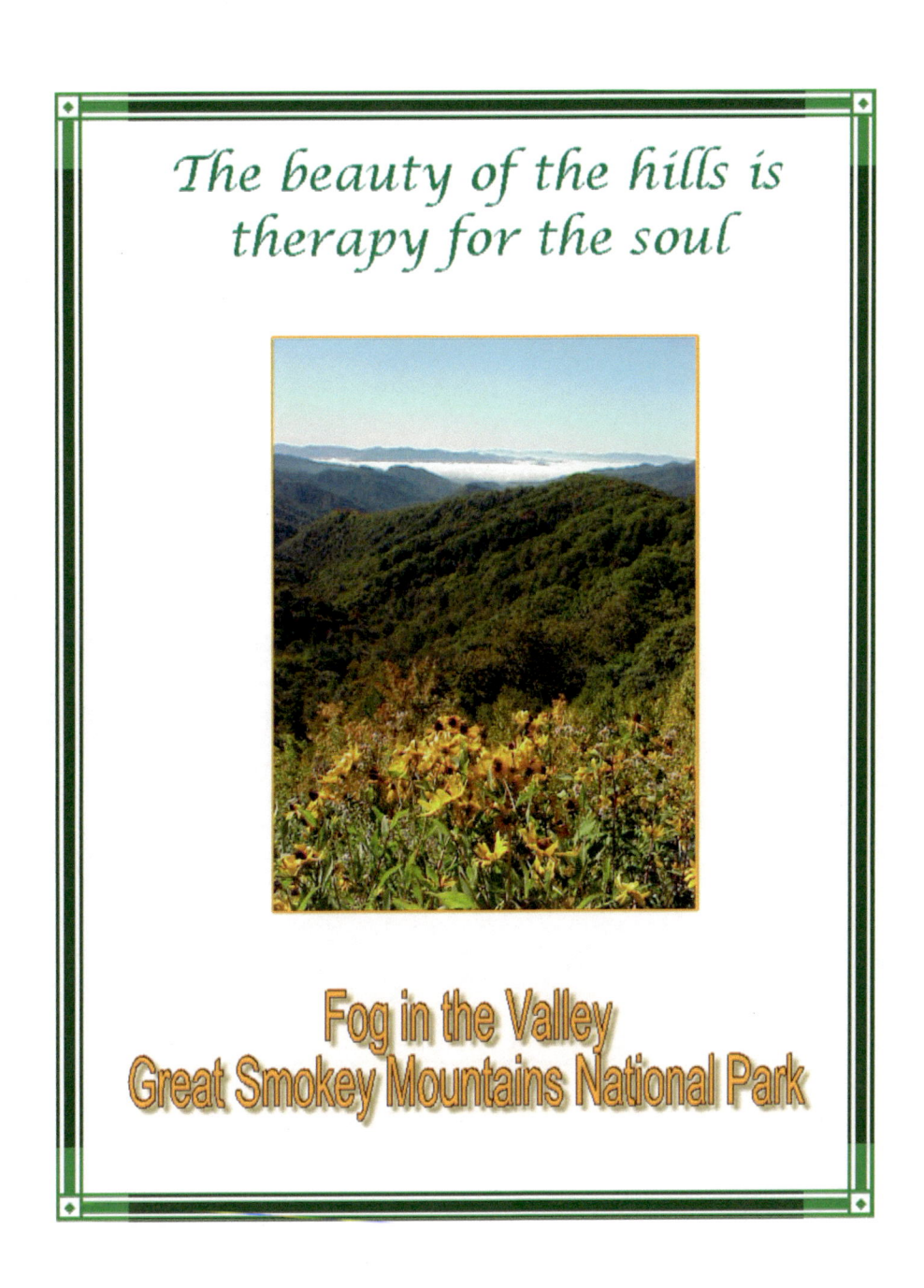

The beauty of the hills is therapy for the soul

**Fog in the Valley
Great Smokey Mountains National Park**

SEASONS

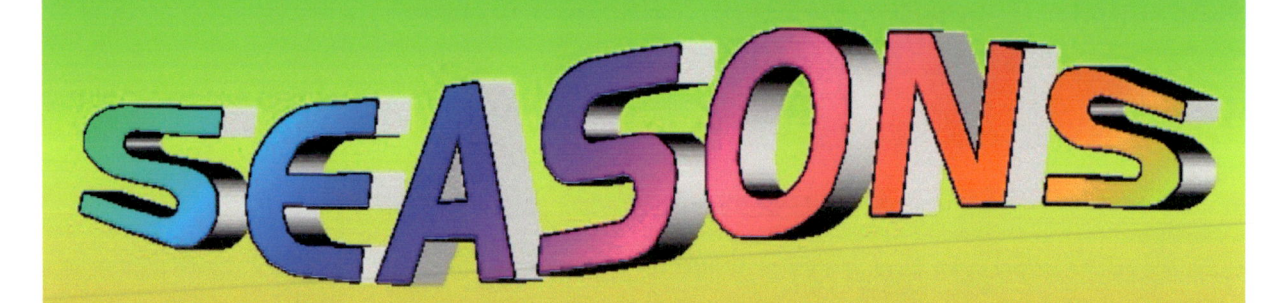

Summer

    Fall

        Winter

            Spring

Beauty supplied by Nature to brighten the day

Celebrating Independence Day

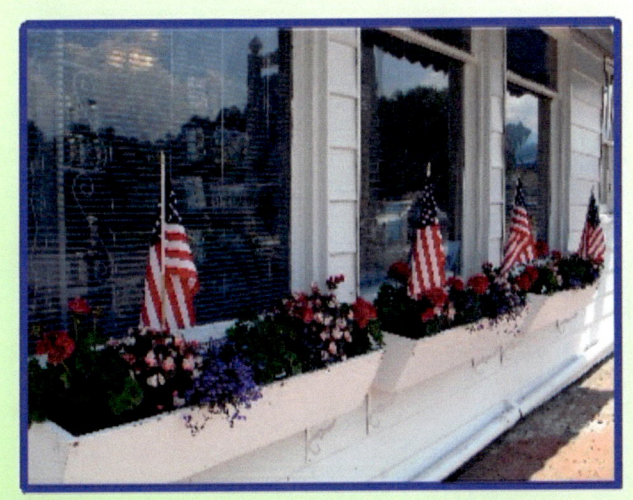

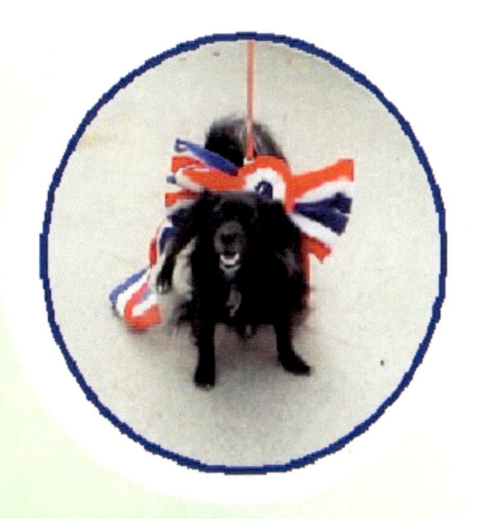

Summer Fun

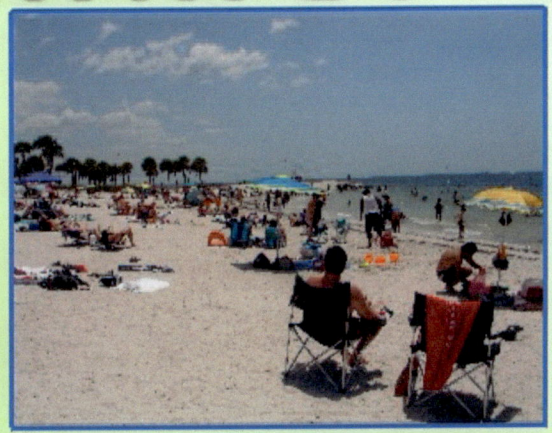

A Day at the Beach

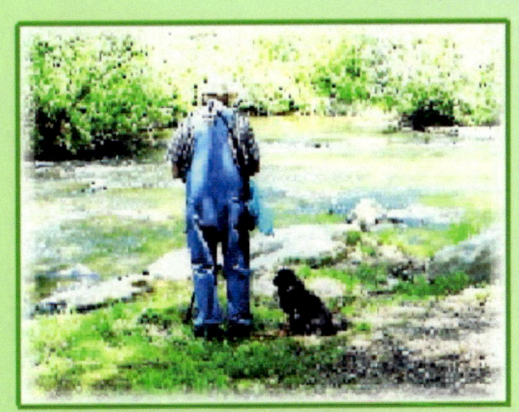

Fishing with a Friend

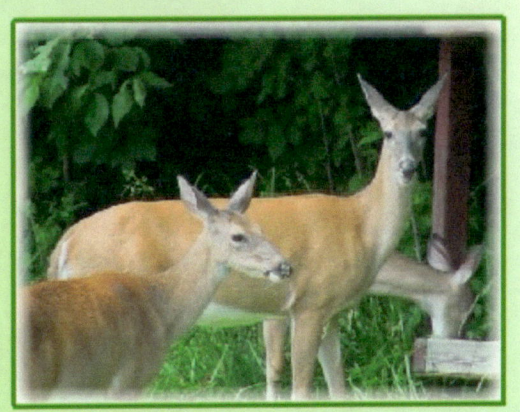

Viewing Nature

Fabulous Fall

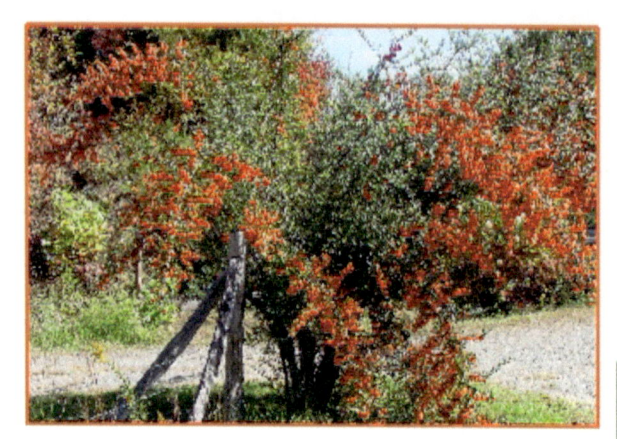

When spirits soar with the crisp fall air and bright colors delight the eyes,
Fall has arrived.

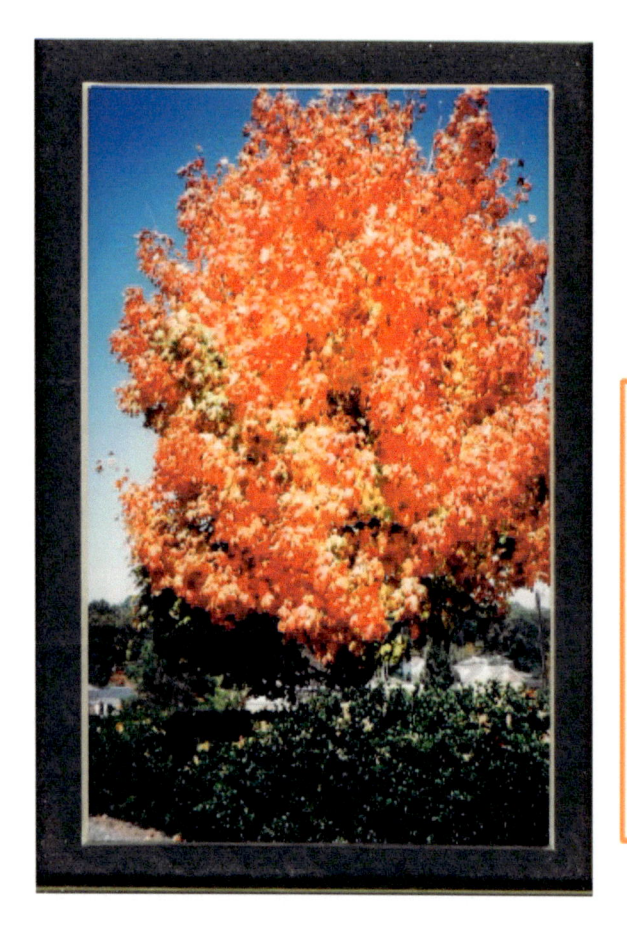

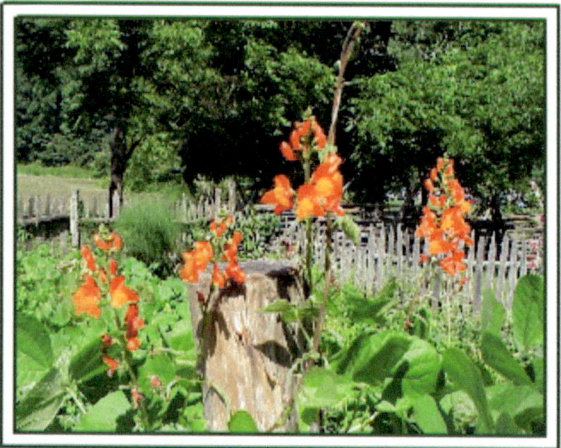

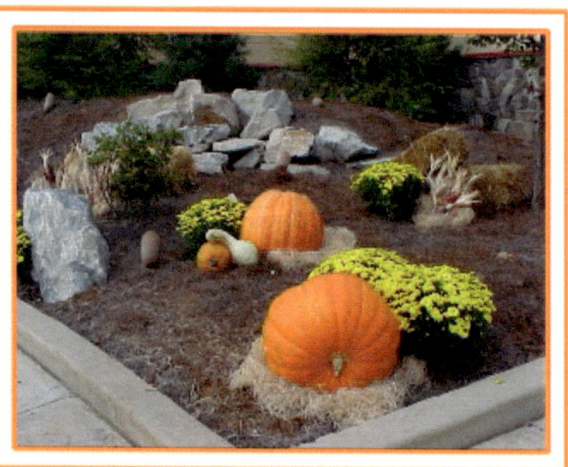

WINTER

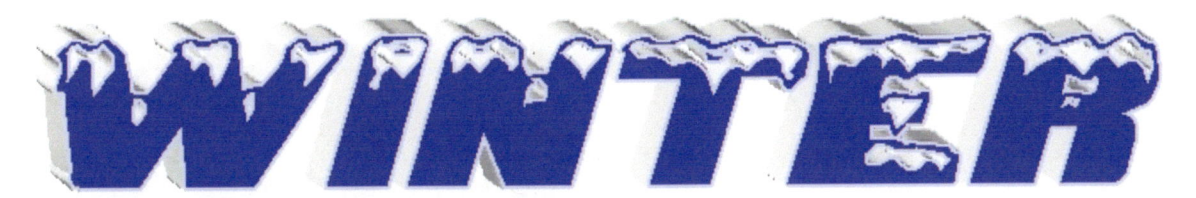

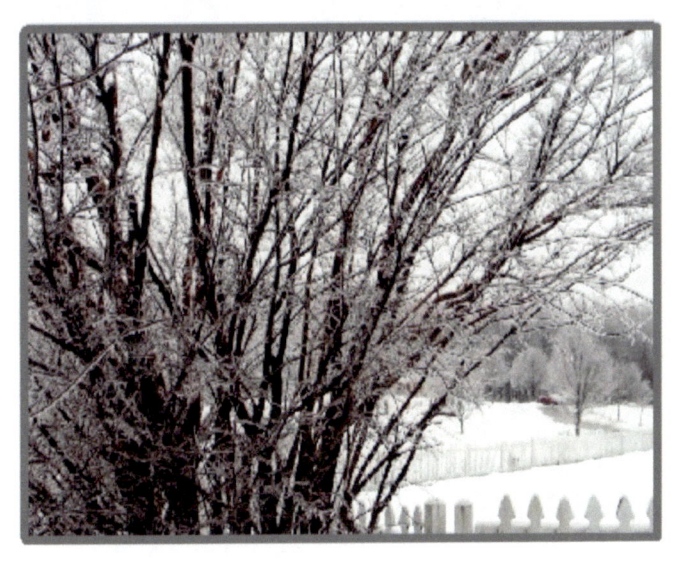

Sparkles and glitter nature provides
putting fine art before our eyes.
The bright sun shines in azure blue skies
while artistic icicles around us lie.
On trees and bushes and lines for power
the beauty lasts for many an hour.
Van Gogh's, Picasso's, DaVinci's so grand
but none so grand as from nature's hand

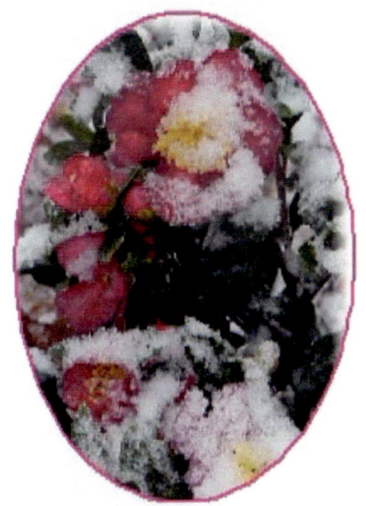

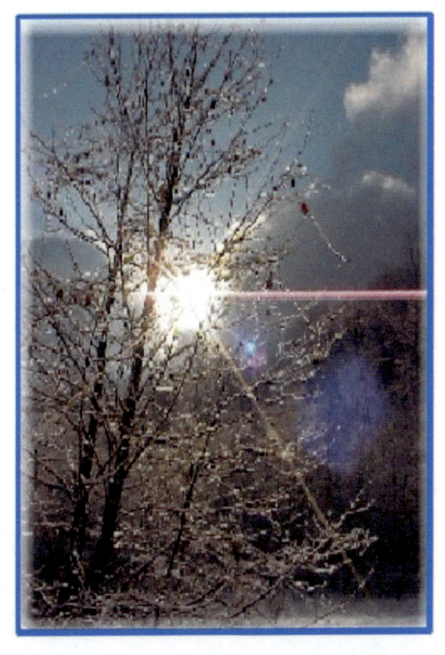

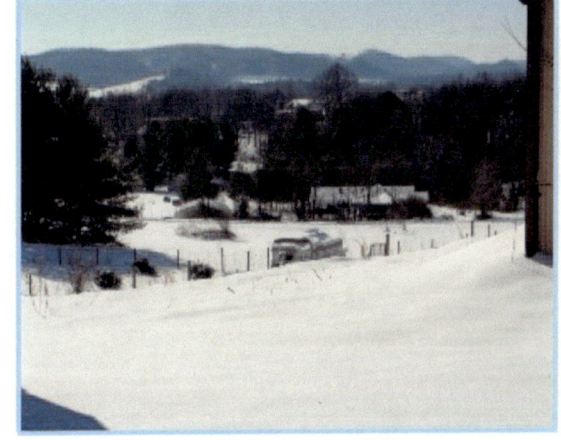

THINK SPRING WILL EVER COME?

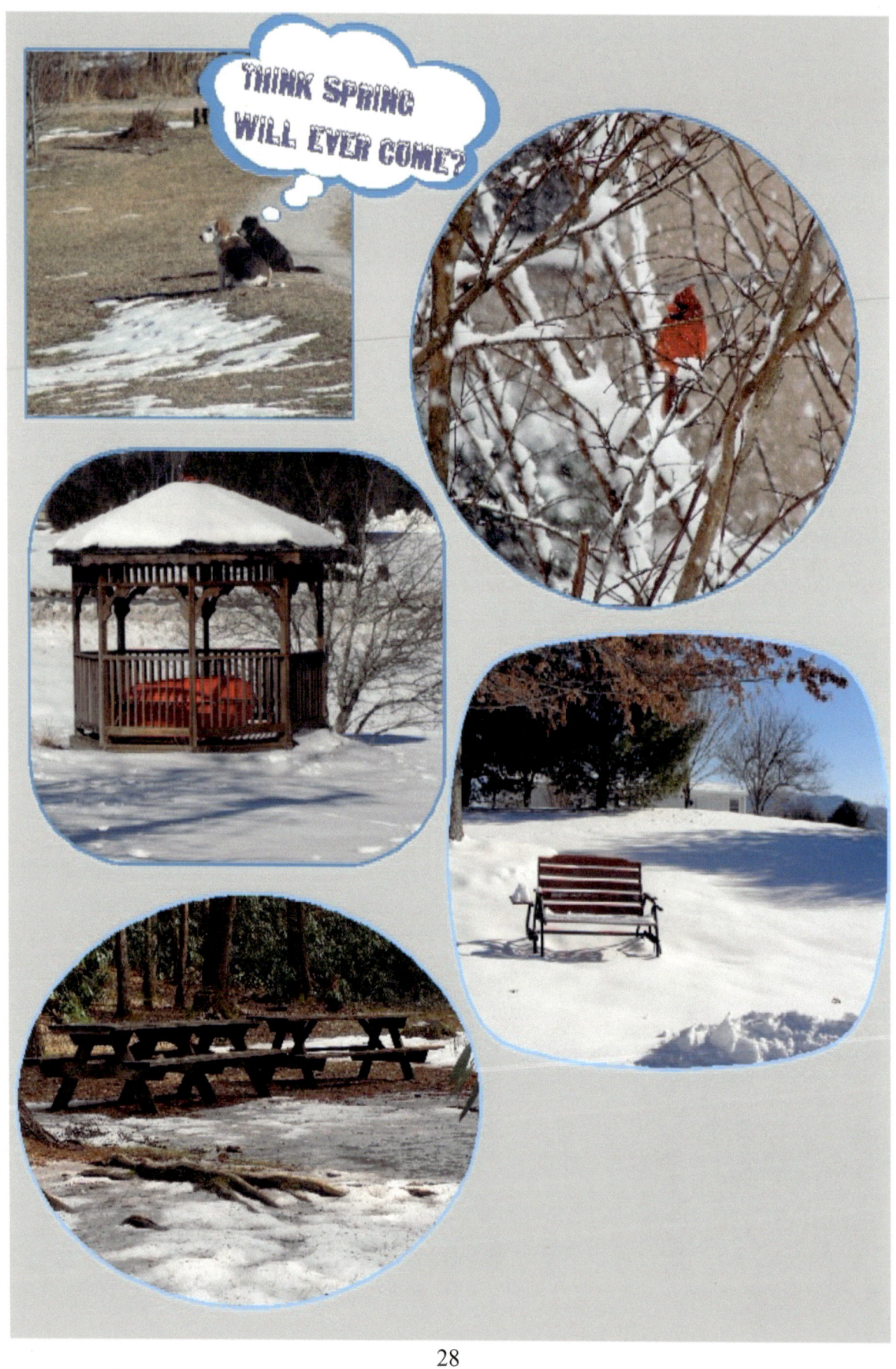

28

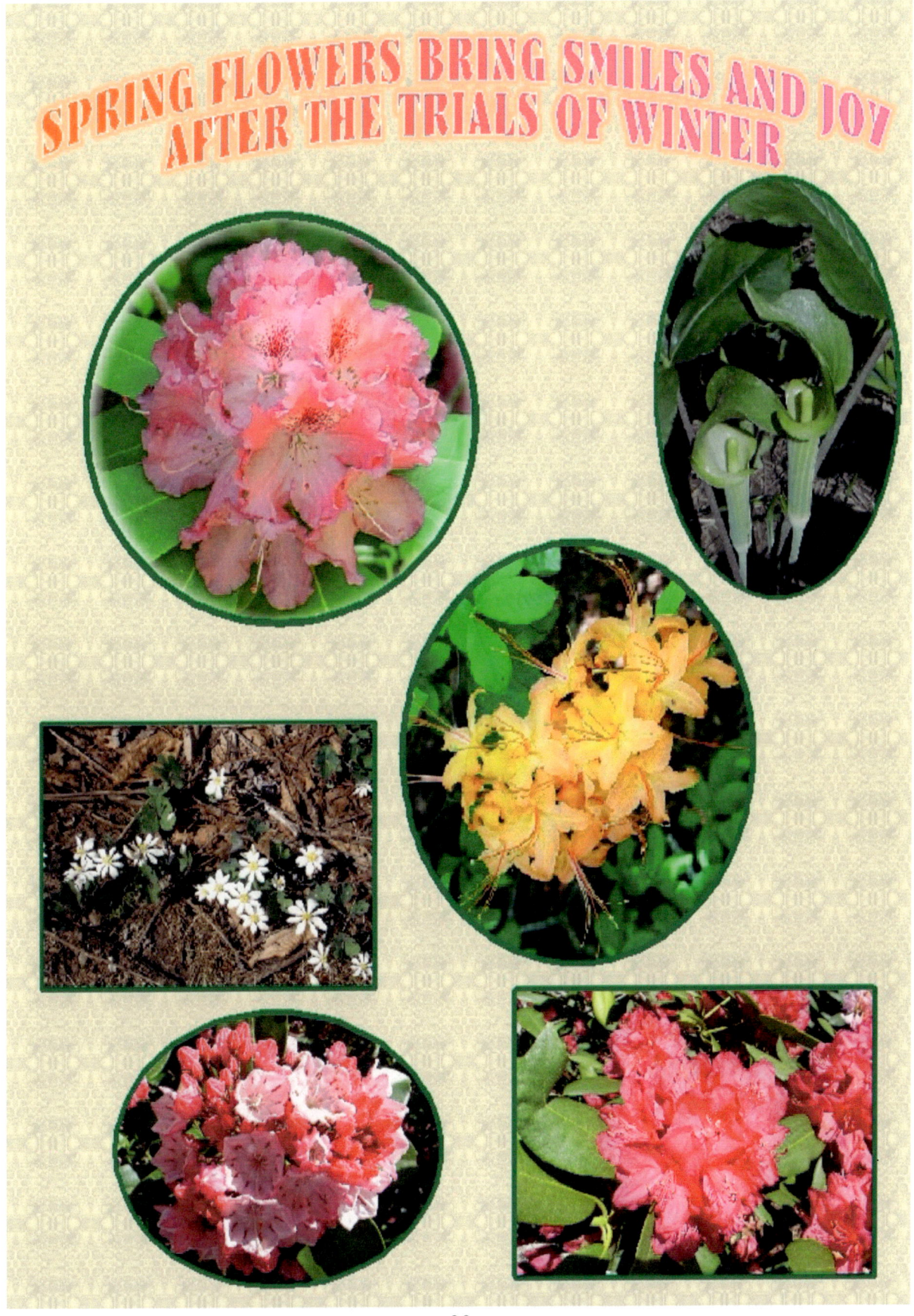

SPRING FLOWERS BRING SMILES AND JOY AFTER THE TRIALS OF WINTER

Summer Splendor

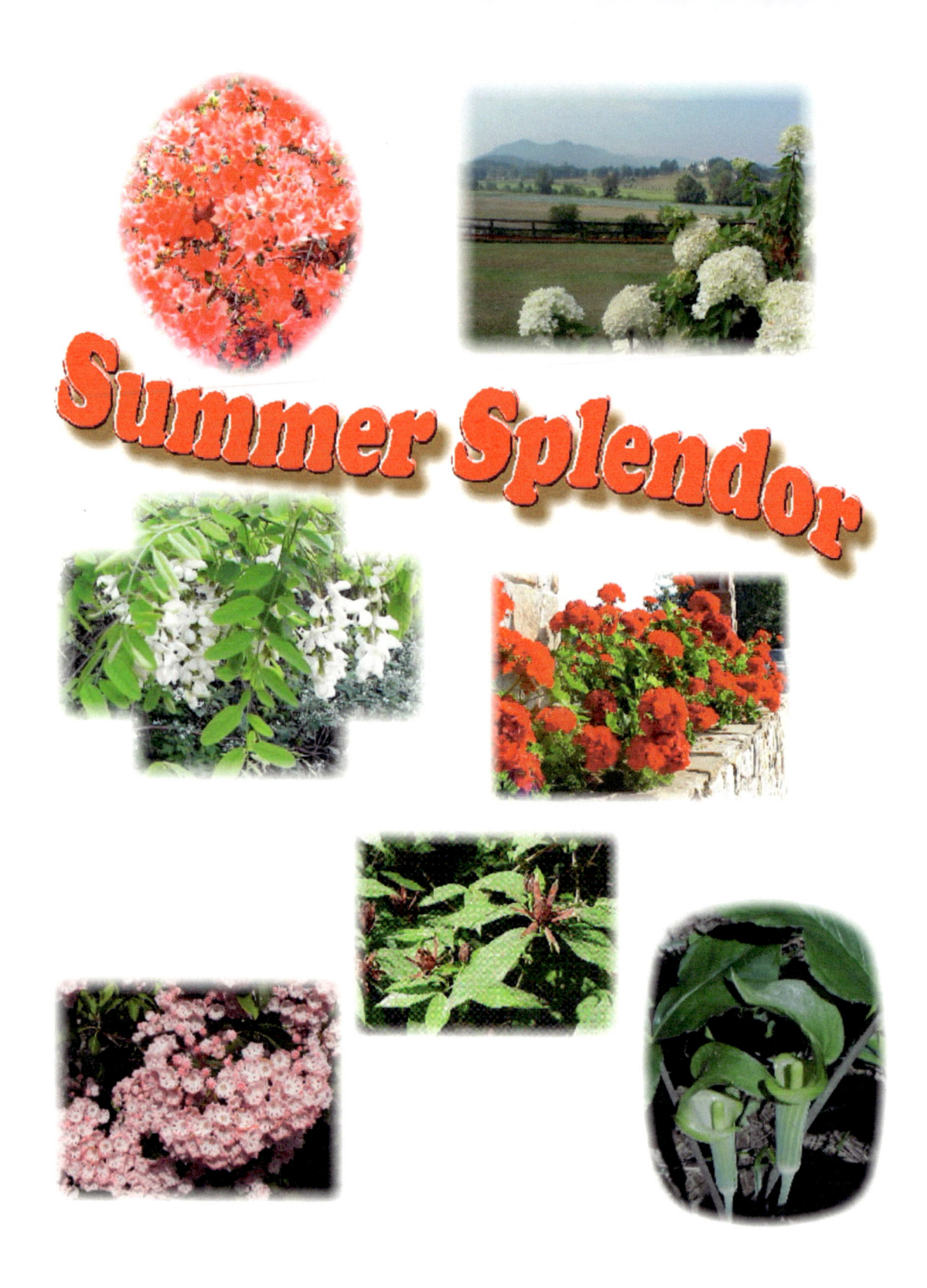

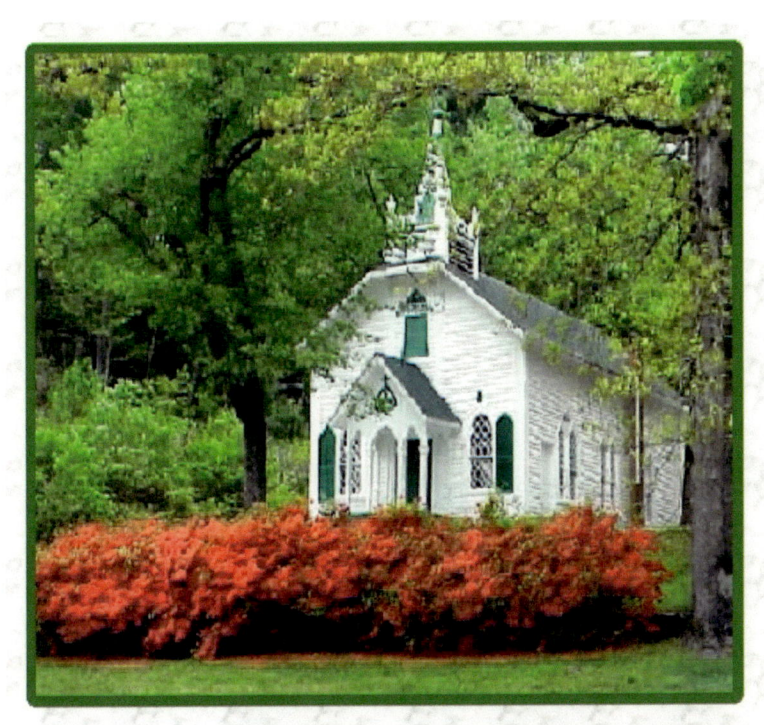

Crescent Hill Baptist Church

Built in 1876, this beautiful little church sits on a hill over looking the beautiful Nacoochee Valley and the Indian Mound in White County, Georgia

SMALL COUNTRY CHURCHES
PLACES OF HOPE, INSPIRATION, AND PEACE

Saint Paul's Episcopal Church

Edneyville,, N.C.

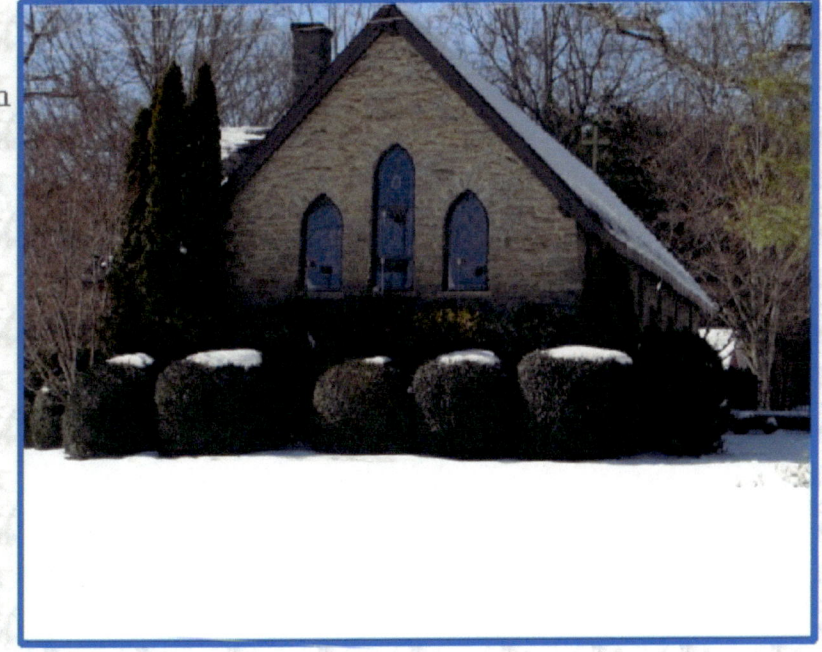

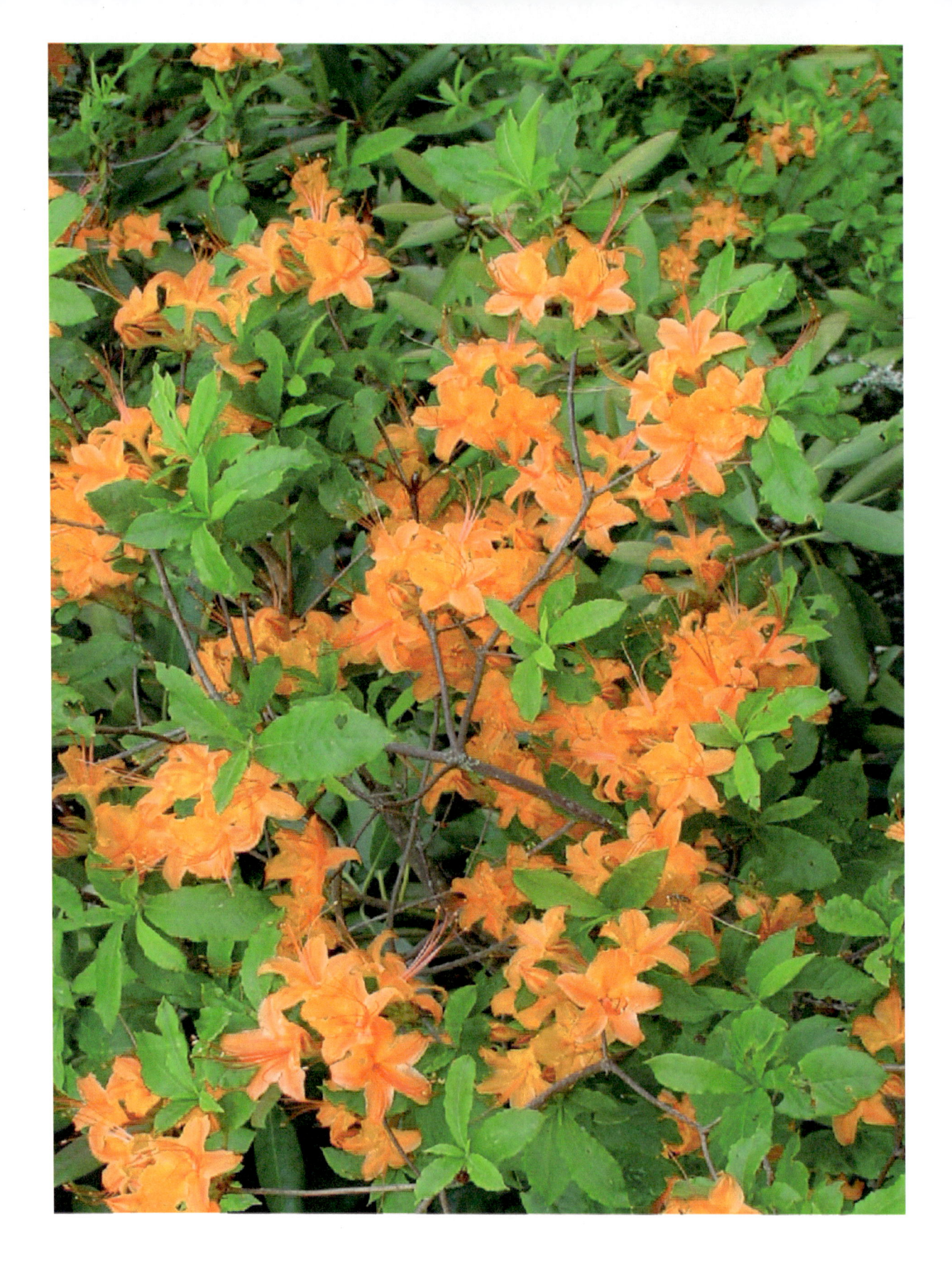

A Day in the Cherry Orchard

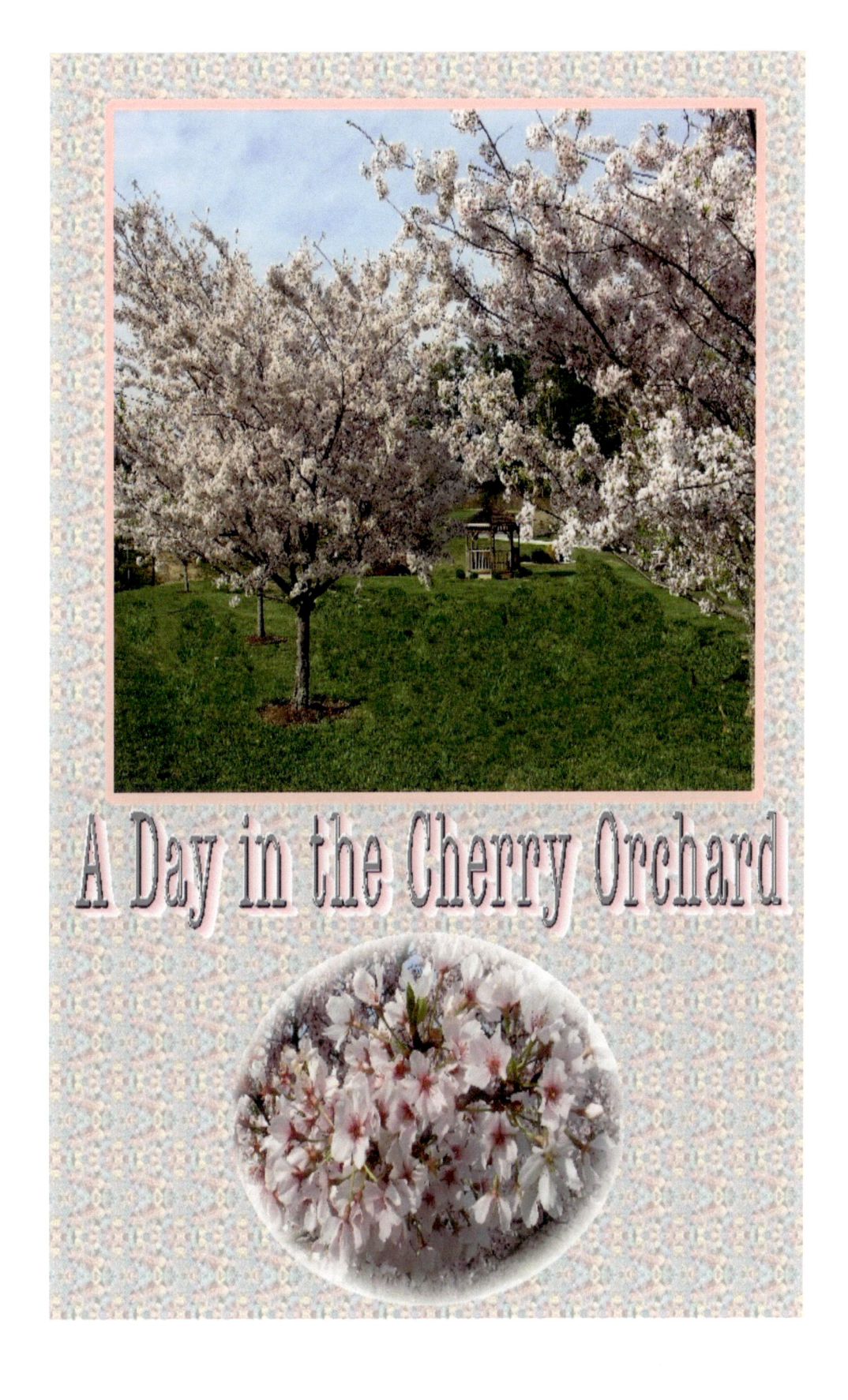

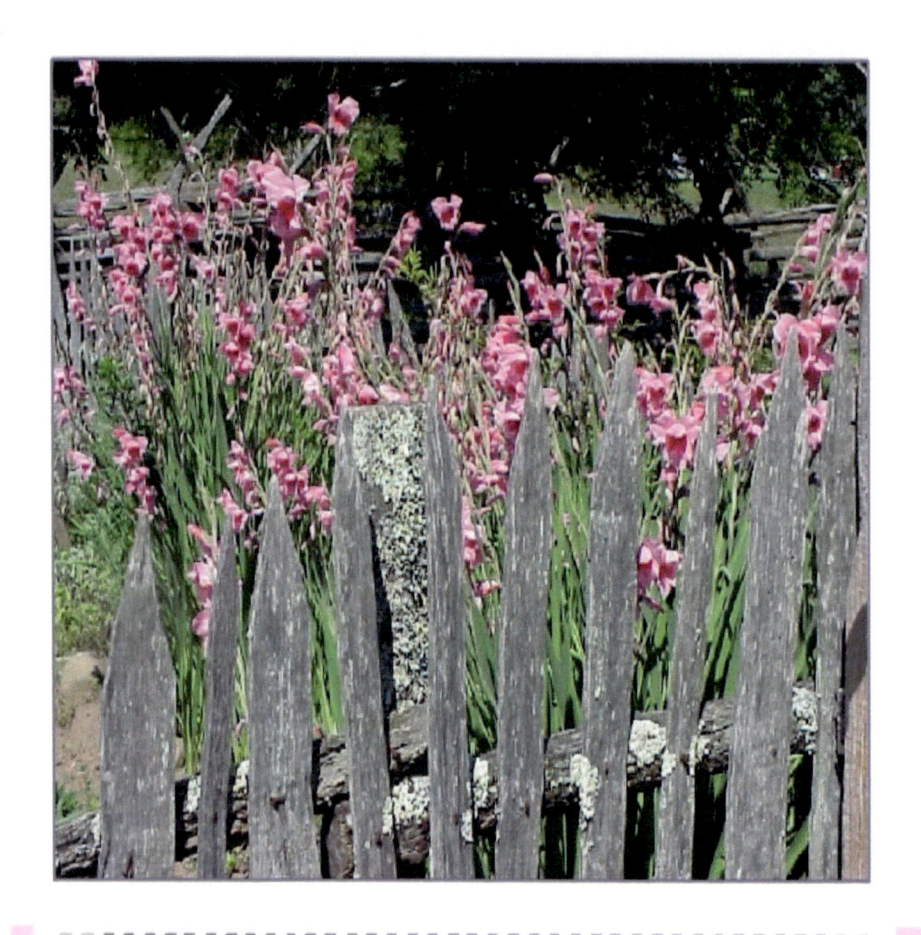

Things to Ponder

Why is the third hand on the watch called the second hand?
If a word is mis-spelled in the dictionary, how would we ever know?
If Webster wrote the first dictionary, where did he find the words?
Why does "slow down" and "slow up" mean the same thing?
Why do "tug" boats push their barges?
Why are they called "stands" when they are made for sitting?
Doesn't "expecting the unexpected" make the unexpected expected?
Why are a "wise man" and a "wise guy" opposites?
Why is phonics not spelled the way it sounds?
Why do we put suits in garment bags and garments in a suitcase?
Why doesn't glue stick to the inside of the bottle?
Why is it a "pair" of pliers when you only have one?
Why is abbreviated such a long word?

IMPORTANT PERSONAL INFORMATION

For security purposes this information can be kept in another location. Make a note on this page where information is kept.

Patient's Legal Name: _____

Also known as: _____

Social Security Number: _____

Spouse's SS Number _____

Medicaid Number: _____

Medicare Number: _____

Military Healthcare Information: _____

_____

Other: _____

_____

_____

Insurance Information:

Company Name – Type Insurance - Policy # - Where policy is kept

_____

_____

_____

Legal Information:

Does anyone have your **power of attorney (attorney in fact)**? Giving someone your power of attorney and making them your attorney in fact means this person can act on your behalf and can make any decision which you yourself can make. There are different powers (general, specific, or health care) which you can bestow on your attorney in fact. A **general** power allows your representative to make decisions for you in *all matters* of health, finance, or otherwise as needed. A **specific** power means that the person can speak for you in only specified situations. A **health care** power allows your representative to make any and all medical decisions for you including medications, treatment, termination of treatments,.etc. when you are unable to do so. *These are important documents to have but be sure to consult a lawyer as to which type meets your needs. Also, be aware that different states have varying laws regarding power of attorney.*

Do you have a Power of Attorney form(s) signed?   Yes _____ No _____
If yes, where is it filed? _____
Who is named as your attorney in fact:
General Power_____

Specific Power_____

Healthcare Power_____

Does your attorney in fact have a copy of the legal document? Yes___ No___
How can your attorney in fact be contacted ?
Name_____Phone_____E-mail _____

_____

Do you have a **Living Will**? Yes_____ No_____ If not, do you want one? Yes_____ No_____
(A living will states your desires regarding treatments and use of medications.)
Where is it filed? _____

Is there a *DNR (Do Not Resuscitate)* order signed?   This is a legal document signed by the patient or their Healthcare Attorney in Fact which stipulates if the patient dies there are to be no efforts to revive them.   Keep this in a place where it can be quickly found.   Doctors, hospitals, and EMTs will need to have a copy of this on file or in hand in case of an emergency.

Are you an **Organ Donor**? Yes___ No___ Where is your card? _____

Do you have a **legal, up to date will**? Yes___ No___
Where is it filed? _____
Who should be contacted about your will?

Name_____ Address_____

Phone_____ Relationship_____

Who is your Executor?_____

Who is your **next of kin**? How can they be contacted?

Name_____Relationship_____

Address_____Phone_____

Who is your **attorney?** How can they be contacted?
Name_____Address_____

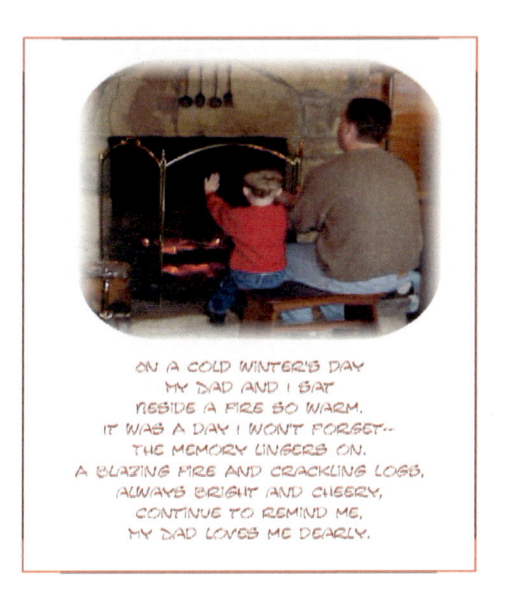

_____Phone_____ Legal Firm_____

*On a cold winter's day
my dad and I sat
beside a fire so warm.
It was a day I won't forget--
the memory lingers on.
A blazing fire and crackling logs,
always bright and cheery,
continue to remind me,
my dad loves me dearly.*

37

Financial Matters

Are there financial matters that need to be checked on?
Does anyone have access to your bank accounts as co-signer, joint tenant, through power of attorney, etc.? Who has this access and how can they be contacted?

Name   Phone   e-mail
_____   _____   _____

_____   _____   _____

Accounts are at which bank(s)?
_____# _____

_____# _____

_____# _____

_____# _____

Are there deposits/withdrawals/auto-pays that need to be seen about?
_____

Are there bills which must be paid on a regular basis? (insurance premiums, house payments, utilities, etc)
_____
_____

Do you have a safe deposit box?   Yes____   No____

Where is it located? _____   Box number? _____

Who is authorized to get into the box? _____

Other information:
_____
_____
_____
_____

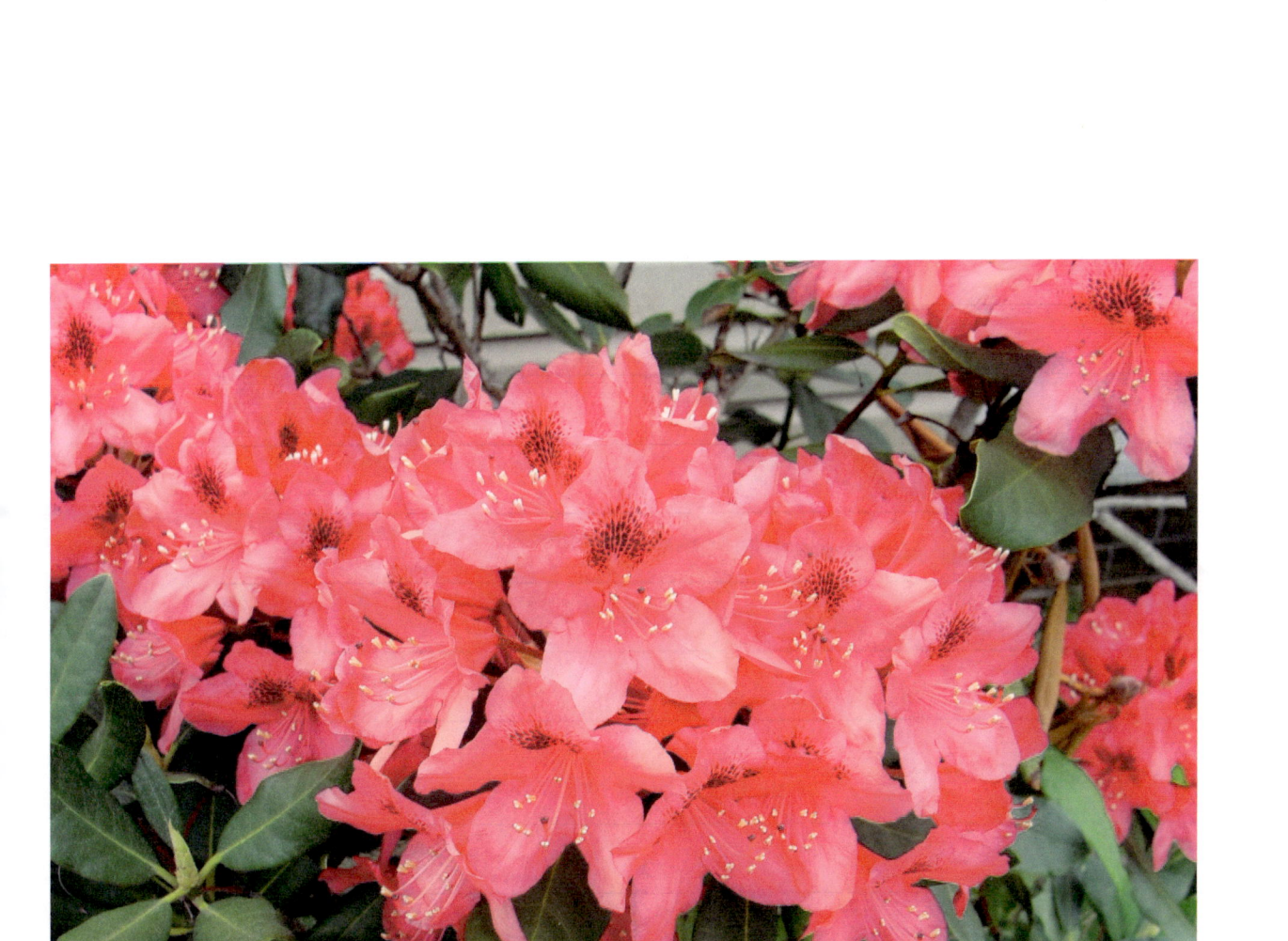

Family Medical History

Make notes about family members who have had medical problems. This may be helpful to your physician in diagnosing or treating illnesses. List diseases, operations, deformities, birth defects, cause of death, age at death, and any other pertinent information.

Great-Grandparents _____

_____

_____

_____

Grandparents _____

_____

_____

_____

Parents _____

_____

_____

_____

_____

Your previous medical history

_____

_____

_____

_____

_____

Your children's medical history
_____
_____
_____
_____
_____
_____
_____
_____
_____
_____
_____

Additional information /comments _____
_____
_____
_____
_____
_____
_____
_____

MEDICATION SCHEDULE CHECKLIST

Enter name of medication required under each day and exact time when it is due.

Mark out the X/time when medication taken.

Morning/Breakfast   Noon   Afternoon/Dinner   Evening/Bedtime   Night

---

Sunday _____

Monday _____

Tueaday _____

Wedmesday _____

Thursday _____

Friday _____

Saturday _____

Sunday _____

MEDICATION SCHEDULE CHECKLIST

Enter name of medication required under each day and exact time when it is due.

Mark out the X/time when medication taken.

Morning/Breakfast   Noon   Afternoon/Dinner   Evening/Bedtime   Night

----

Sunday _____

Monday_____

Tueaday_____

Wedmesday_____

Thursday_____

Friday_____

Saturday_____

Sunday_____

MEDICATION SCHEDULE CHECKLIST

Enter name of medication required under each day and exact time when it is due.

Mark out the X/time when medication taken.

Morning/Breakfast   **Noon**   **Afternoon/Dinner**   **Evening/Bedtime**   **Night**

Sunday _____

Monday_____

Tueaday_____

Wedmesday_____

Thursday_____

Friday_____

Saturday_____

Sunday_____

MEDICATION SCHEDULE CHECKLIST

Enter name of medication required under each day and exact time when it is due.

Mark out the X/time when medication taken.

Morning/Breakfast   Noon   Afternoon/Dinner   Evening/Bedtime   Night

---

Sunday _____

Monday _____

Tueaday _____

Wedmesday _____

Thursday _____

Friday _____

Saturday _____

Sunday _____

MEDICATION SCHEDULE CHECKLIST

Enter name of medication required under each day and exact time when it is due.

Mark out the X/time when medication taken.

Morning/Breakfast   **Noon**   **Afternoon/Dinner**   **Evening/Bedtime**   **Night**

Sunday _____

Monday _____

Tueaday _____

Wedmesday _____

Thursday _____

Friday _____

Saturday _____

Sunday _____

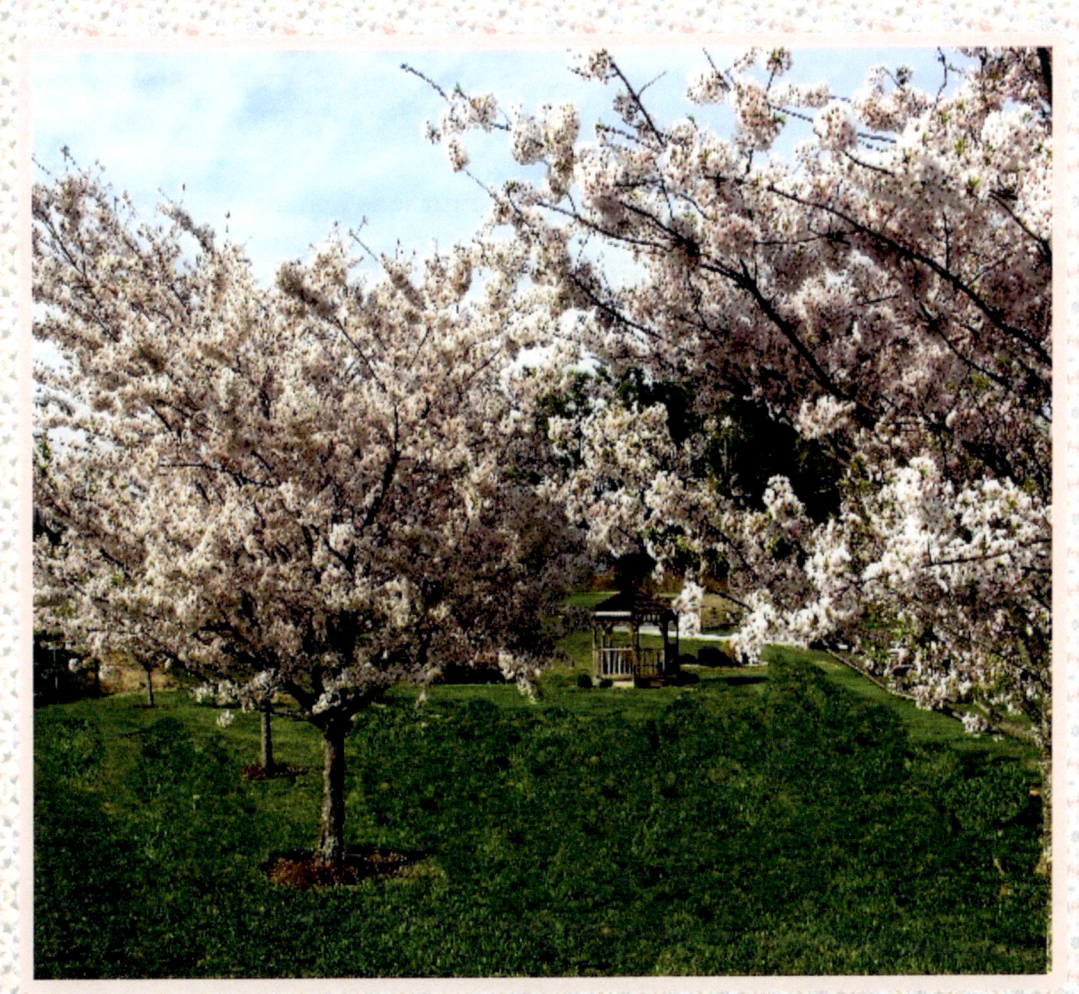

A Day in the Cherry Orchard

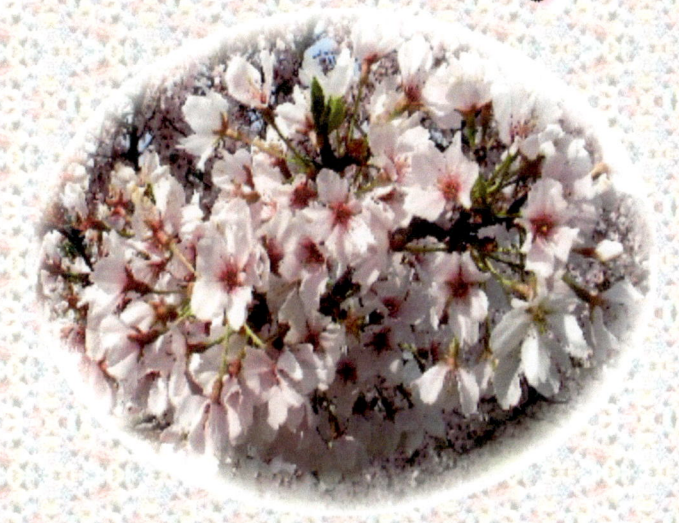

MEDICATIONS

Be aware that all drugs have side affects. As few as 3 medications can cause drug interactions. Always discuss medications and their effects with your doctor and/or pharmacist.

Medication Name /Phone/ Fax/E-mail	Prescribed by	RX #	# Refills	Instructions/warnings/ Allergic reactions	Pharmacy Druggist

MEDICATIONS

Be aware that all drugs have side affects. As few as 3 medications can cause drug interactions. Always discuss medications and their effects with your doctor and/or pharmacist.

Medication Name	Prescribed by /Phone/ Fax/E-mail	RX #	# Refills	Instructions/warnings/ Allergic reactions	Pharmacy Druggist

DAILY MEDICAL DIARY

Make additional copies of this form and keep the completed forms in this book for reference and to follow progress

Day/Date/Time---Blood Pressure/Pulse/Temperature/Medication---Comments-------Doctor/Nurse

_____
_____
_____
_____
_____
_____
_____
_____
_____
_____
_____
_____
_____
_____
_____
_____
_____
_____

Notes:

_____
_____
_____
_____

DAILY MEDICAL DIARY

Make additional copies of this form and keep the completed forms in this book for reference and to follow progress

Day/Date/Time---Blood Pressure/Pulse/Temperature/Medication---Comments-------Doctor/Nurse

_____
_____
_____
_____
_____
_____
_____
_____
_____
_____
_____
_____
_____
_____
_____
_____
_____

Notes:

_____
_____
_____
_____

DAILY MEDICAL DIARY

Make additional copies of this form and keep the completed forms in this book for reference and to follow progress

Day/Date/Time---Blood Pressure/Pulse/Temperature/Medication---Comments--------Doctor/Nurse

_____
_____
_____
_____
_____
_____
_____
_____
_____
_____
_____
_____
_____
_____
_____
_____

Notes:

_____
_____
_____

DAILY MEDICAL DIARY

Make additional copies of this form and keep the completed forms in this book for reference and to follow progress

Day/Date/Time---Blood Pressure/Pulse/Temperature/Medication---Comments-------Doctor/Nurse

_____
_____
_____
_____
_____
_____
_____
_____
_____
_____
_____
_____
_____
_____
_____
_____

Notes:

_____
_____
_____
_____

DAILY MEDICAL DIARY

Make additional copies of this form and keep the completed forms in this book for reference and to follow progress

Day/Date/Time---Blood Pressure/Pulse/Temperature/Medication---Comments--------Doctor/Nurse

_____
_____
_____
_____
_____
_____
_____
_____
_____
_____
_____
_____
_____
_____
_____
_____
_____
_____
_____
_____
_____
_____

Notes:

_____
_____
_____
_____

EMERGENCY CONTACTS

EMERGENCY ASSISTANCE: Ambulance, Emergency Medical Technicians (EMT's)
911

Ambulance: PHONE:_____

Fire Department: PHONE:_____

Police Department PHONE:_____

Doctor:_____Nurse_____

Phone:_____Cell phone:_____E-mail/Fax:_____

Doctor:_____Nurse:_____

Phone:_____Cell phone:_____ E/mail/Fax:_____

Doctor:_____Nurse:_____

Phone:_____Cell phone:_____ E/mail/Fax:_____

Doctor:_____Nurse:_____

Phone:_____Cell phone:_____ E/mail/Fax:_____

Pharmacy:_____Pharmacist_____

Phone_____E-mail_____

Medications_____
_____
_____

Hospital:_____

Address:_____

Phone:_____ Fax:_____ E-Mail:_____

Personal Contacts:

Family:

Name	Phone	Cell phone	E-Mail/Fax

Friends –Ministers-other important contacts:

Name (relationship)　　　　　　Phone　　　　　　　Cell phone　　　　　　　E-Mail

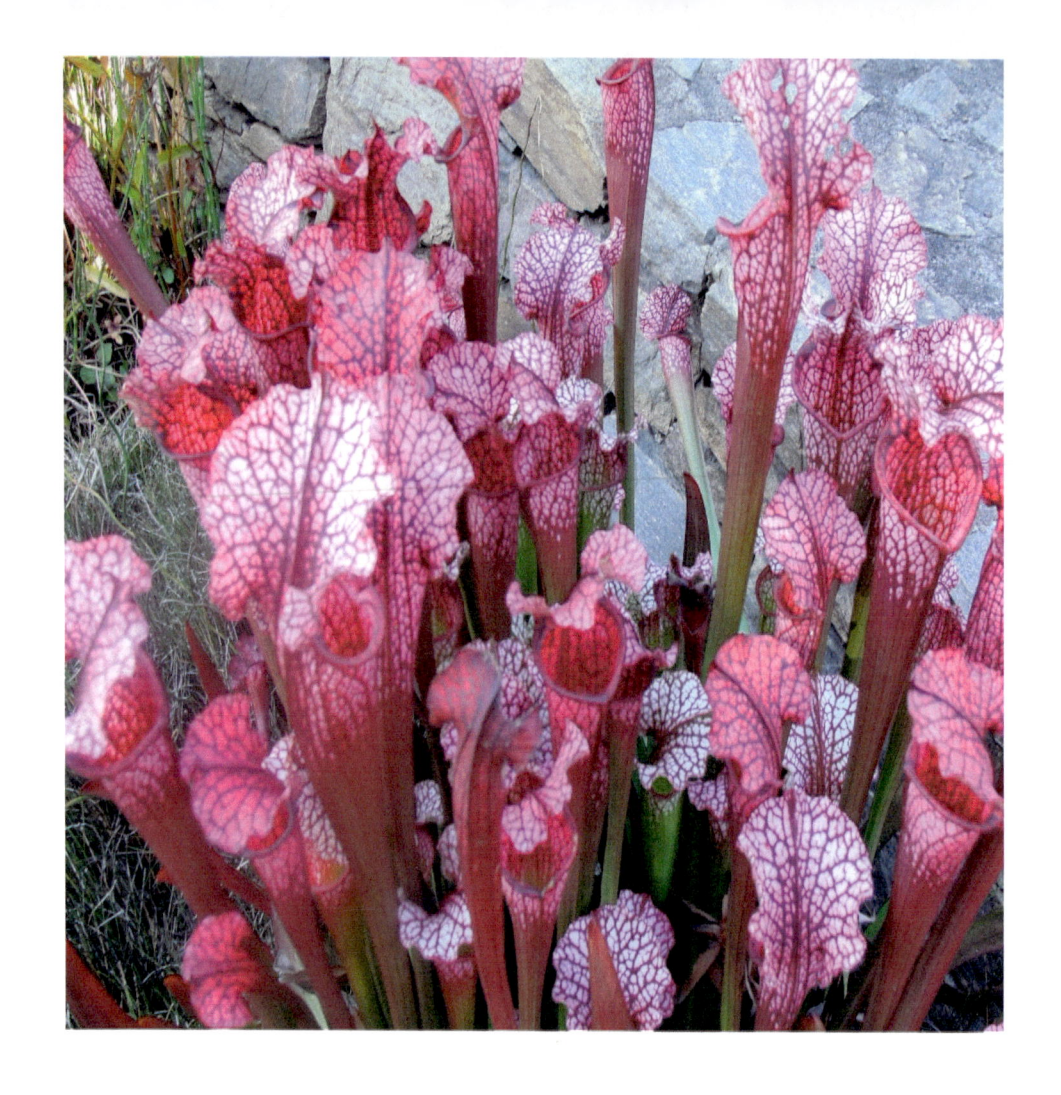

January_____

_____
February_____

_____
March_____

_____
April_____

_____
May_____

_____

June_____

_____

July_____

_____

August_____

_____

September_____

_____

October_____

_____

November_____

_____

December_____

_____

Have a calendar (preferably in a book that can always go with you) to keep information about medical schedules, appointments, notes about special happenings, and MILEAGE to medical services. Mileage can often be a tax deduction.

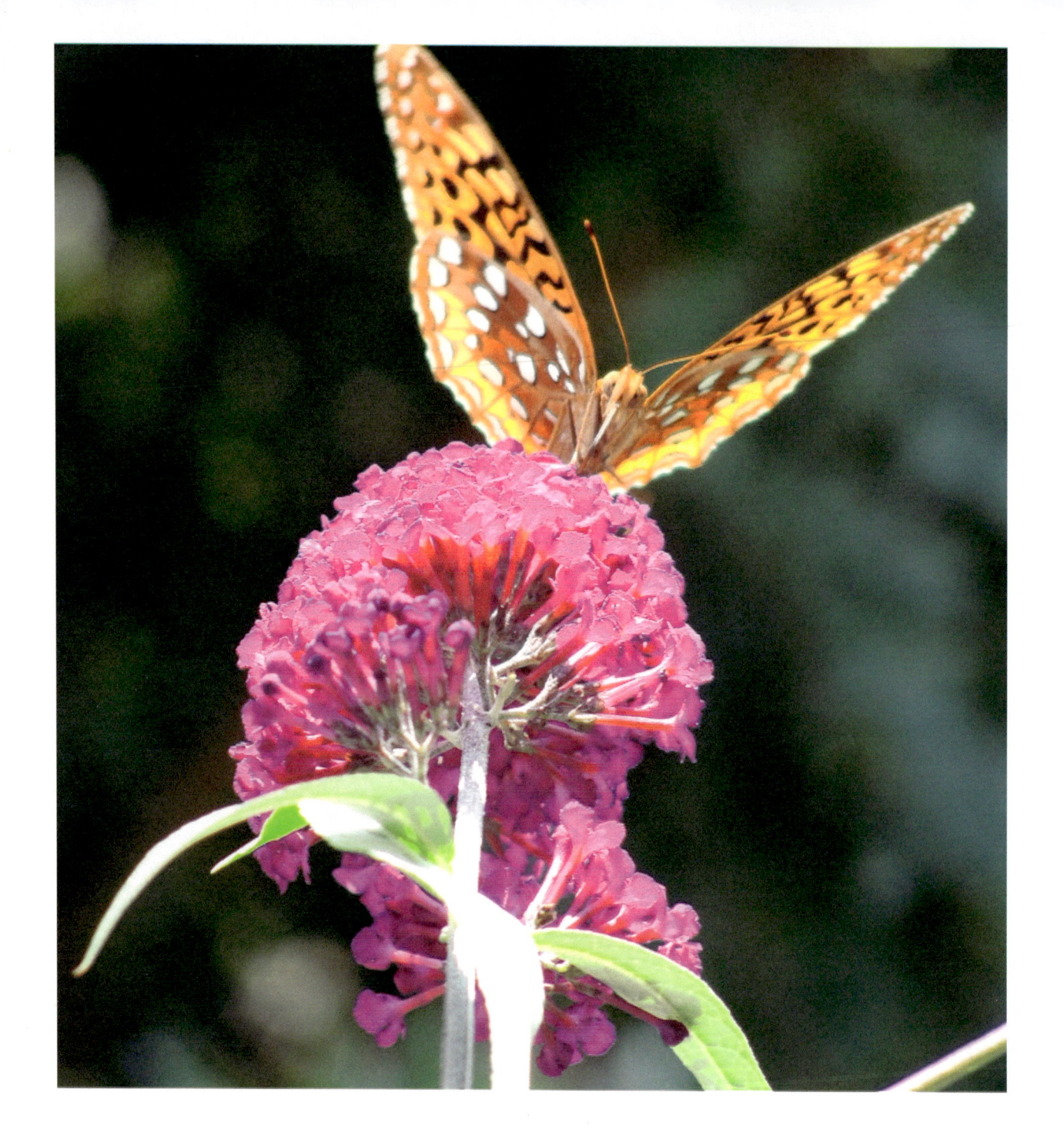

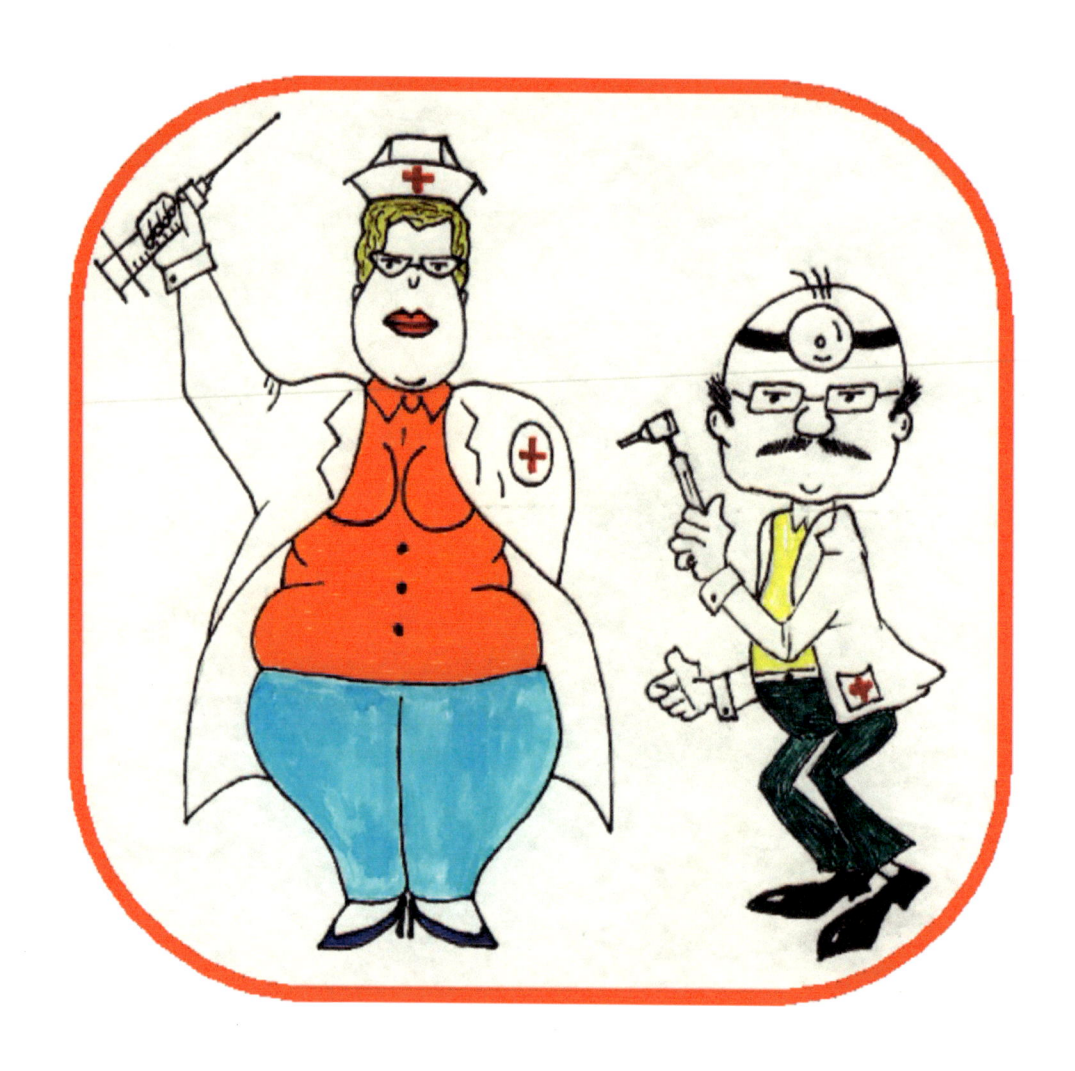

The staff wishes you and yours the best, and good health. No matter what happens, always look
Toward Better Days.

Made in the USA
Columbia, SC
05 July 2024